Healthy Green Recipes

from

Around the World

by

Stephanie Grey

Disclaimer : This information is presented by a registered nurse but for informational purposes and not to be used to diagnose or treat diseases or illnesses. See your Primary Care Physician for any illnesses or health concerns you have and feel free to share material in this book with them.

Cover Design by Create Space
ISBN -13 : 978-1490937946
ISBN-10 : 1490937943
Volume 1
Printed in USA
Published by Create Space

Preface

We are becoming a very diverse society each day and so we should learn about the cultures that surround us. A great way is through foods and beverages, and we all can learn from each other. Through learning foods from other countries, we also learn about the people and how we all have differences and similarities, weaknesses and strengths, poverty and riches. This book is created to do just that, to help us understand other cultures through what they eat and drink.

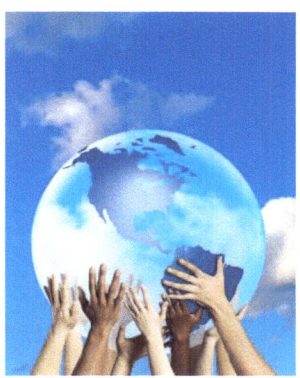

We didn't get all nations, but a sample of recipes from around the world, will open your world and help you appreciate them as well. We will be doing more cookbooks as we gather more recipes from our friends across the globe, so feel free to send them to **snursegrey@aol.com**. We are focused on holism and healthy living, and recipes are not limited to food, but to healthy lifestyles, in homes, workplaces, community and environment. House cleaning tips, clean air, clean water, safe workplaces, reducing toxins in our environment, are all a part of our focus. Our cookbooks are geared towards helping us take better care of ourselves and our planet Earth, as God wants:

" Beloved, we wish above all things,

that you prosper and be in health,

even as thy soul prospereth."—3 John 1:2

Acknowledgements

- Special thanks to God, and His knowledge and my experience of His presence, in helping me write and publish this book to promote health and help prevent illnesses.

- We also thank my mom, son, siblings and relatives, who all taught me how to cook in many times through out my life and being able to share that with all we serve.

- We also thank the many non-profits, businesses, nursing/medical schools, healthcare facilities I have worked or been a patient of, government agencies and faith-based communities who have imparted knowledge over the years to help me share that with the world.

- We thanks, most of all, those we are called to serve, locally, nationally and globally, to help them promote health and prevent diseases (mental, physical, spiritual), in their communities God has placed them.

Contents

Chapter 1 : Introduction

Our world has become very diverse, in communities and nations, and sometimes we cannot visit other countries, but through preparing meals, we can have a touch of them. I have been in USA and Canada, but have tried many dishes from across the globe and hence my reason, to share some with you. I have met people from across the globe as well, and learnt a lot from them, and also from studying various nations and their cultures. This cookbook have many recipes and nations include : Jamaica, USA, Canada, Middle East, India, and Mexico . This is our first edition, and our next volumes will include more nations and cultures. So please enjoy these recipes, as I have tried some, and share with others as well. Reading this book and also trying some of the recipes, will help you become more culturally sensitive and learn to understand and appreciate the various cultures on God's precious land.

Allow your children to try some, with supervision of course, and we do have a special chapter just for them, with dental health, food safety and hygiene information as well. I have personalized the book, giving it a more interesting read, and also makes the recipes and food come more alive. We believe food is medicine, and exercise as well, and through out the book, you will learn a holistic approach to not only food, but everyday life, to enhance your well-being. Share information in your home, community and churches/places of worship, and lets all move toward a healthier future together!!

Chapter 2 : Jamaican Recipes

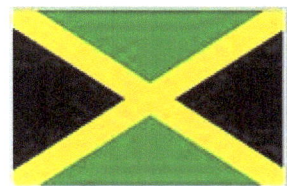

JACK MACKEREL CASSEROLE

Ingredients :

Mackerel in Brine**, Sweet potato(cooked and crushed)*

2 boiled eggs, Milk, Cinnamon, Vanilla

Sauté the following and place in casserole dish :

Vegetable oil, Onion(rings) , Olives, garlic(crushed), Tomato, sweet pepper

Directions :

Spread flaked mackerel over sweet potato in dish. Add sautéed vegetables. Add pinch of salt and pepper to taste, Layer grated cheese(cheddar),Sprinkle Brown sugar. Broil for 350F – 10 mins.

**Substitute Meat with Fish /Tuna and also Yam/Dasheen/Green Banana for Sweet Potato.

CREAM OF CAULIFLOWER SOUP

Ingredients : 2 cups cauliflower, ½ cup chopped onion, 1 cup water, 2 tbs. butter, 2 tbps. flour, 1 can coconut milk, ¼ tsp. salt, 1/8 tsp. black pepper, ¼ tsp. curry powder.

Directions : Simmer the above until tender- 20 mins., Puree in electric blender. Heat butter and blend in flour and cook until lightly browned. Add coconut milk stirring until smooth. Mix in puree, salt, pepper and curry powder.

Did You Know ???

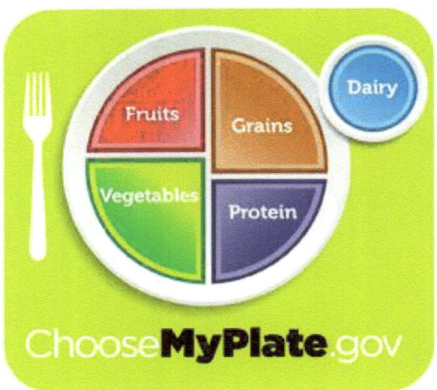

This is the new nutritional guide which has replaced the Food Pyramid and hopefully, the obesity rate will decrease. Visit **www.choosemyplate.gov** and join the movement!

THREE BEAN SALAD

Ingredients : 1 can 16oz Green beans, 1 can red kidney beans

1 cup chopped. Celery, 4 scallions (chopped)

1 cup chopped bell pepper (red, yellow, orange), ½ cup chopped. Dill pickle

¾ cup vinegar and oil dressing, ½ tsp. Salt, 1/8 tsp. black pepper

Directions : Mix all ingredients, then chill and serve.

WALDORF SALAD

Ingredients : 4 Med. Sized tart apples- diced, ¾ chopped Celery,1/3 cup chopped. Walnuts, ½ cup raisins, ¾ cup coconut mayonnaise, Lettuce leaves. *Directions* : Mix all ingredients and serve on a bed of lettuce.

POTATO SALAD

Ingredients : 2 lbs. red potatoes, 1 small onion, ½ cup finely chopped dill pickle, ¼ cup vinegar and oil dressing, 1 tsp. salt, 1/8 tsp. pepper, ½ cup coconut mayonnaise, 1 medium celery stalk chopped, 2 hard-boiled eggs coarsely chopped.

Directions : Chop potatoes into ½ inch cubes and cook in boiling water until tender. Drain water and let cool. Mix with potatoes. Cover and chill.

FRUIT AND COCONUT SALAD

Ingredients : 1 ½ cups chopped fresh pineapple, 2 bananas, sliced 2 oranges, peeled and diced, 2 apples, cored and diced, 1 cup raisins/ chopped dates, ½ cup shredded coconut, ¾ cup coconut mayonnaise, Lettuce leaves.

Directions : Mix all ingredients together and serve immediately.

COCONUT ORANGE PANCAKES

Ingredients : 1 cup flour, 1 ½ tsp. baking powder, ¼ tsp. salt, 1 ¼ cup orange juice¼ cup grated coconut, 1 egg, 1 tbsp. molasses.

Directions : Mix first four ingredients and then mix the rest and then combine together.

COCONUT BRAN MUFFINS

Ingredients : 1 cup water, 1 tbs. vanilla extract, ½ cup honey, 1 egg, ¼ cup wheat bran, 1 cup flour, ¼ cup grated coconut, 2 tsp. baking powder, ¼ tsp. salt, 1 tsp. cinnamon, ½ tsp. nutmeg, 3 tbsp. Melted butter, ½ cup nuts.

Directions : Combine first five ingredients and let sit for 10 minutes, then mix next remaining. Preheat oven to 400 degrees. Add melted coconut oil to liquid ingredients, add nuts and dry ingredients and mix together until moist. Do not over mix, pour into greased muffin cups. Bake 15 minutes, yield 12.

BEETROOT SALAD

Ingredients : 4 Medium Beet roots (roasted/boiled and chopped into bite-size pieces) ½ cup chopped hazel nuts-toasted, extra virgin olive oil, 1 navel orange segmented, 1 navel zest and juice, Salt and pepper to taste.

Directions : Drizzle on extra virgin olive oil, then top with Parmesan Cheese.

AVOCADO RICE

Ingredients : 1 Cup Basmati rice- cooked, 1 Avocado- chopped in bite size pieces. Extra Virgin Olive Oil, salt and pepper to taste, chopped parsley, lime juice.

Directions : Combine, and serve immediately.

SNOW PEAS AND WATERCHESTNUTS

Ingredients : 2 cups snow peas, 1 can water-chestnuts, salt and pepper to taste .Sesame Seeds-optional, Soya sauce, Cornstarch, Red pepper flakes.

Directions : Stir fry and serve topped with sesame seeds.

VINAIGRETTE

Ingredients : Dijon Mustard, grated shallots/onions, honey/brown sugar, celery salt. Red wine vinegar, ground pepper.

Directions : Combine and store in covered tight jar.

MEATLOAF

Ingredients : Ground beef/turkey/chicken, Chopped Onions, Chopped garlic, Oregano, Bread crumbs, Oats, Salt and Pepper to taste.

Directions : Shape into Loaf, Bake 35 mins. Top with Tomato Sauce, Brown Sugar, Butter. Bake 10 mins. at 400F. Remove from oven and rest. Slice and serve with: Noodles, Cream Potatoes and a salad. Recipes courtesy of ***PAMRY DLIGHTS AND CATERING,*** by **Miss Paulette Grey (Jamaica, West Indies).**

Tropical Fruit Salad by Stephanie Grey

Ingredients : 1/2 cup diced watermelon, 1/2 cup diced cantaloupe, 1/2 cup diced peaches, 1/2 cup fresh blueberries, 2 tablespoons of vanilla yogurt and 1/2 tsp. cinnamon

Direction : Combine all ingredients together , mix gently and serve right away. Great for summer months !

Jamaican Curried Chicken by Mrs. B.I. Grey

Ingredients : 1-2 pounds of grain-fed Chicken (you can use whole or breast with bones, thighs, legs and wings), salt and pepper to taste, 1-2 tbsp. curry powder, 2 medium carrots chopped, 1 medium red onion or 2 sprigs of escallions, tomatoes, canola oil (remember chicken has its own fat), and herbs of your choice.

Directions : Sauté onions or escallions in canola oil and add curry powder, but don't burn. Cut chicken in small pieces and wash then add. Cook for 30-45 minutes of moderate heat and then place on low to simmer. Add tomatoes, herbs and salt to taste. You can serve over cooked rice and beans/peas or with sweet potatoes, dumplings and yam, or green banana. Eat also with tossed salad with greens and lemonade, on the side as well.

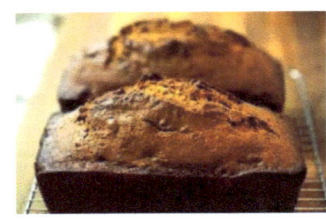

Pumpkin Bread   by Stephanie Grey

Ingredients : 2 eggs, 1 ½ cups sugar, 1 cup pumpkin smashed after cooking or 1 can, ½ cup oil or plant-based butter, ½ cup water, ¼ tsp. baking powder, dash of salt, ½ tsp. cloves, ½ tsp. cinnamon, 1 2/3 cup flour, 1 cup crushed almonds, walnuts or pecans.

Directions : Sift and mix flour, baking powder, sugar, cinnamon, cloves and salt. Mix butter, sugar and pumpkin separately and water. Mix dry and wet ingredients and stir until smooth. Place in oiled bread tin and top with crushed walnut, pecans or almonds. Bake in oven at 350 degrees until ready and serve warm with fruit salad and tea or coffee of your choice!

Sugar-Free Pumpkin Biscuits by Stephanie Grey

Ingredients : 2 cups whole wheat flour, ½ cup natural stevia sugar,1 tbsp. baking powder, ½ teaspoon salt, 1 teaspoon ground cinnamon, ½ teaspoon nutmeg, ¼ teaspoon ginger, 6 tablespoons cold, light vegetable butter, cubed, ¾ cup canned pumpkin or boiled and mashed,¼ cup fat-free milk or almond or soy milk, 1 large egg or 1 cup egg white

Directions : Heat oven to 400 degrees and place liners in muffin cups. Mix all dry ingredients : stevia sugar, baking powder, salt and spices and then add cubed cold butter an mix until crumbly. In another bowl whisk pumpkin, milk and egg and then fold into dry ingredients and mix until mixture is smooth then add to each muffin cup, 2/3 full, leaving space to rise. Brush top with oil and sprinkle crushed walnut or pecans, your choice. Bake for 20 minutes.

Ginger-Mint Tea : Get some grounded or raw grated ginger and a mint-tea bag or fresh mint. Place in a teapot and pour boiling filtered water. Steep for about 5-10 minutes and sweeten with sugar of your choice. Good for indigestion, nausea , diarrhea and vomiting.

Tamarind Drink : Remove pulp of tamarind from seed and hull, by pouring hot water and leave for 12-24 hours. Strain and sweeten to taste, with stevia or brown sugar. Serve over crushed ice, great in summer! *Ginger Beer* : Get some raw ginger, wash thoroughly, then mash and place in a pot of boiling water. Remove from heat and leave over night. Drain and sweeten to taste with brown or sugar-free stevia in the raw. A must for every kitchen pharmacy!

Chapter 3 : Americas & Canada

MANGO BREAD

Ingredients : 2 cups all-purpose flour, 2 teaspoons baking soda

1 teaspoon baking powder & 2 teaspoons cinnamon

3 eggs, well beaten, 3/4 cup canola oil

1 1/2 cups granulated sugar, 2 cups peeled and diced fresh mango

1/2 cup raisins, 1/2 cup macadamia nuts chopped

1/2 cup grated coconut

Directions : Preheat oven to 350°F. Grease and flour two 9x5 inch loaf pans. Sift the flour, baking soda, baking powder and cinnamon into a small bowl. In a large mixing bowl, combine eggs, oil and sugar mix with dry ingredients until well blended. Fold in mango, raisins, nuts and coconut. Pour into loaf pans and bake 45 to 50 minutes or until a toothpick inserted in the center come out clean. Let cool 10 to 15 minutes, take out of pans and let completely cool on baking tray enjoy .

Recipe sent from **Diane Grey, Toronto, Canada**

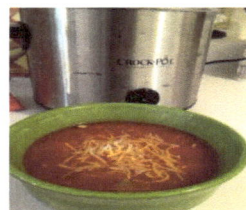

Heart Healthy Bean Chili   **By Kori Burton**

Ingredients : -2 cups chopped onion, -1 1/2 cup chopped peppers (red, yellow, orange, and green mix), -1 cup chopped carrots, -2 cloves of garlic finely chopped, -16oz vegetable broth, -1 1/3 cup canned crushed tomatoes-1 cup canned diced tomatoes in juice, -1 can kidney beans, -1 can northern beans, -1 cup of corn, -1 teaspoon oregano, -1 teaspoon ground cumin-1 teaspoon ground chili powder. *Directions* : Cook in crockpot medium-high heat for 4 hours.

English Blueberry Muffins

Ingredients : -1 beaten egg, -1 cup of skim milk, -2 tsp. lemon juice

-1/4 cup vegetable oil, -1/4 cup of sugar, -3 tsp. baking powder

-1 cup or more of freshly picked blueberries

Directions : Cook at 425 for 25 minutes or until golden tops

By Kori Burton

Orange Almond Chocolate Cake

Ingredients : -1 1/2 cup flour, -1 tsp. baking powder, -1/3 cup unsweetened baking cocoa, -1/2 cup sugar, -1/2 cup almond milk, -1/2 cup orange juice, -2 tsp. vanilla extract, -2 tbsp. balsamic vinegar.

Directions : Preheat oven to 375. Sift Dry ingredients into 9x9 pan. Whisk wet ingredients (except vinegar) into pan. When batter is consistently smooth, mix in the vinegar. Bake for 30 minutes.

***Almond Frosty** : -1 cup almond milk, -1 tsp. cocoa, -1/8 cup chopped almonds, -1/2 cup ice

Directions : Blend until smooth. **Sincerely, Kori Burton**

Smokey Greens

Ingredients : 3 bunches of turnip greens, 3 bunches of mustard greens, 1 cup water, 1 tablespoon extra virgin olive oil, 4 cloves garlic, minced, ½ cup red onion, diced, 1 large dried smoked pepper, 2 tablespoons apple cider vinegar, fresh ground black pepper and salt to taste as desired.

Directions : 1. Wash and trim greens. 2. Heat oil in a large stockpot over medium heat. Add onion and garlic and sauté for 3 minutes or until onion is soft. 3. Add smoked pepper, vinegar, salt and pepper. 4. Cover, reduce heat to medium low and simmer for 1 hour. Stir every 15 minutes and add more water if necessary. Season with salt and pepper to taste.

Prep Time : 10 minutes **Cook Time** : 1 hour **Serving Size** : ½ cup **Nutrition Facts (per serving)** : calories : 68/ Total Fat : 2 grams / Saturated Fat : 0 / Sodium : 70 mg / Carbohydrate : 5 grams / Fiber : 3 grams / Protein : 2 grams

Source : Church Health Center Wellness Education, visit **www.chreader.org** for more recipes.

Oven Fried Chicken

Ingredients : ½ cup cornmeal, ½ cup panko breadcrumbs, 1 tsp. dried tarragon, 1 teaspoon dried basil, 1 teaspoon dried oregano, ¼ tsp. salt, ¼ tsp. black pepper, ¼ tsp. ground red pepper, 1 teaspoon onion powder, 1 teaspoon garlic powder, 4 egg whites, ¼ cup low fat butter milk, ½ cup whole-wheat flour, sifted, 6, 4-ounce boneless chicken breasts, Cooking spray.

Directions :

1. Preheat oven to 375 degrees.
2. 2. In a shallow pan, combine cornmeal, breadcrumbs, tarragon, basil, oregano, salt, black pepper, red pepper, onion powder and garlic powder.
3. In another shallow pan, combine the egg whites and buttermilk.
4. In a third shallow pan, place the flour.
5. Coat the chicken with flour, dip in egg mixture, then roll in cornmeal mixture.
6. Place in a large glass baking dish coated with cooking spray.
7. Bake uncovered for 18 minutes or until chicken is no longer pink in tender and juices run clear.

Prep Time : 10 minutes **Cook Time** : 18 minutes **Serving Size** : 1 chicken breast

Nutrition Facts (per serving) : Calories : 225/Total Fat : 2gms/ Saturated Fat : 1 gram/

Sodium : 275 mg/ Carbohydrate : 22 grams/ Fiber : 1 gram/ Protein : 30 grams

Source : Church Health Center Wellness Education,

visit **www.chreader.org** for more recipes.

Chapter 4 : Asia and the Middle East

Now, let's take you to the Middle East and Asia, where we will sample recipes from Asia, India, Israel and Iran. They will make you feel like, you're really there !!

India : Beet Soup

Ingredients : 4 beetroots, peeled and grated, 1-2 cups of Basmati rice

1 Tbsp. Butter, 1 cup water, add more if needed, grated cheddar cheese (optional).

Directions : Peel and grate beetroot, then melt butter in a large pan. Add grated beetroot and basmati rice and cook. Add water, then salt and pepper to taste. Serve with cheese grated and/or butter.

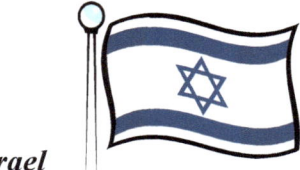

Israel

There are seven fruits commonly used by Israelites : wheat, barley, grapes, figs, pomegranates, olive oil and dates. Yael Eckstein, says :

> *" each one of the Seven fruits of Israel represent a unique*
>
> *attribute of God and deserves a special berakhah*
>
> *(blessing) to be recited over them." (Eckstein, 2012).*

Here are some of her recipes.

Barley is a great grain used from in Biblical days and it was seen as food for poor people and also used to feed cattle and livestock. It is very beneficial to one's health, in blood glucose stabilization, cardiovascular health and cancer prevention.

Coconut Milk Cream of Barley Soup

Ingredients : 1 cup pearl barley, rinsed thoroughly, 1 onion chopped, 1 carrot sliced, 2 celery ribs sliced, 2 bay leaves, 4 sprigs fresh parsley, 1 tablespoon chicken soup powder, salt and freshly ground black pepper, 1 cup coconut milk/cream, 1 tablespoon canola oil and 5 cups water.

Directions : Sauté vegetables in oil for 5 minutes, stir occasionally. Combine all ingredients except the coconut cream in a pot and bring to a boil over high heat. Reduce the heat and simmer covered until the barley is tender. 1 to 1 ½ hours. Add the coconut cream and heat.

Pomegranate Salad

Ingredients : 1 (10 ounce) package mixed baby greens or fresh spinach, 1 pomegranate, peeled and seeds separated, 1 (8 ounce) package crumbled feta cheese, 1 small cucumber, chopped Chopped scallions or red onion (optional).

Dressing :

Ingredients : 1 cup mayonnaise, 2 tablespoons mustard, 1 1/2 tablespoons honey, 1/2 tablespoon lemon juice , salt and pepper to taste. *Directions* : Combine all ingredients and place on salad above. (Eckstein, 2012).

Fruit Salad

Ingredients : 1 apple, 1 bundle of grapes, 1 pear, 1orange, 5 figs, 5 dates, 1 cup of pomegranate seeds, 1/2 teaspoon of cinnamon.

Directions : Chop all of the fruits, put together in a big bowl, top with cinnamon.

Author : Eckstein, Y. (2012). *Seven fruits of Israel : Recipes and Devotions from the Holy Land.* Booklet, from the International Fellowship of Christians and Jews, pgs.

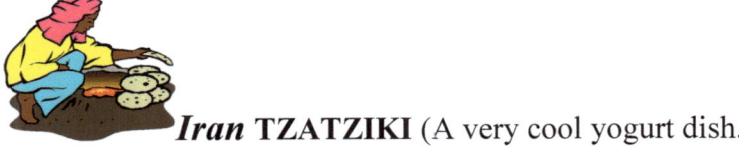 *Iran* **TZATZIKI** (A very cool yogurt dish.

This is a great recipe from the Middle East !

Ingredients : ½ cucumber , basil and fresh mint leaves, yogurt, extra virgin olive oil, garlic cloves chopped, lemon juice, turmeric, dash of salt to taste.

Directions: Chop basil and mint leaves and cube cucumbers. Add mixture to yogurt and stir to combine. Add salt, tumeric, extra virgin olive oil, garlic and lemon juice to taste. Serve right away, great in summer months.

Falafel by Stephanie Grey, my personal version!

Ingredients : 2 Tbsp. flour, 2 cups carrots, 1 cup sunflower seeds, 1/3 cup ground flax seeds, 1 cup fresh parsley, 3 tbsp. onion, diced, 1 clove garlic, dash of salt, ½ tsp. ground cumin, ½ tsp. curry powder, ½ cup sesame seeds.

Directions : Process carrots to a paste and add sunflower seeds, flax seeds, garlic and spices. Add onion and parsley then stir in sesame seeds. Roll a tbsp. each into balls, dehydrate for 2-3 hours and then fry in oil or bake on oiled baking sheet. Serve with Mediterranean Salad. The **Mediterranean Diet** has also proven to be very healthy because of the amount of vegetables, fruits, garlic, olive oil that's used in it's dishes. They all enhance immunity and great for heart health, especially in lowering cholesterol. High in fiber, low in saturated fats and sugar, making use of natural oils and sugars from plants . You should at times try some recipes and remember to also keep physically active and manage stress as well. It's good in both prevention of diabetes, cancer and heart disease/stroke, and also in the treatment of these conditions as well.

Chapter 5 : Children Recipes !!

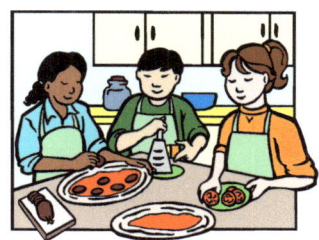

We created this section especially for the little ones and youth as well. It also has important tips for parents or caregivers of children and youth. Obesity, cancer, diabetes, foodborne illnesses and safety are areas of interest for all children and youth.

Food safety is very important , especially when cooking with your children. Close supervision is needed, and many children have become victims if burning from stove cooking and/or fires, some with injuries that are permanent needing much plastic surgery. Teach them how to properly wash their hands, here's a cool recipe :

> *1. Wet hands with warm water, but if not available,*
>
> > *cold water is okay.*
>
> *2. Lather bath hands with soap.*
>
> *3. Scrub hands for at least 15-20 seconds.*
>
> *4. Rinse hands thoroughly.*
>
> *5. Dry hands on a clean towel.*
>
> *Recipe for Protection and Health by Stephanie Grey*

(1) A prayer a day, keeps the devil away, so pray God's Word daily over your child/youth and family. (2) Teach your child to pray simple prayers, like Psalm 23 and John 3:16 !

(3) Be an example of health for your child/youth, 3 John 1:2 & Romans 12: 1-2.

Apple Crisp by Stephanie Grey

Ingredients : 4 large apples, ¾ cup stevia sugar, ½ cup flour, 1 tsp. cinnamon,1 ½ cup rolled oats 1/3 cup butter (non-airy).

Directions : Heat oven to 350 degrees and then peel apples, core and slice them. Toss with ½ cup stevia, 1 tbsp. flour and cinnamon. Spread on baking sheet and then mix other rolled oats with flour and sweetener and then add butter until crumbly. Sprinkle evenly over fruit and bake until browned.

Healthy Pizzas by Stephanie Grey

Ingredients : Use whole-wheat English muffins, bagels or pita bread as the crust. Have tomato sauce, low fat cheese and cut up vegetables or fruits for toppings.

Directions : Let kids help and select their favorite ingredients. Place in oven to warm and serve with healthy drinks like low calorie lemonade (see below)

Low Calorie Lemonade by Stephanie Grey

Ingredients : 1 quart filtered water, 1-2 lemons or 4 packs true lemon. 1 cup stevia sugar, 1 tray of ice cubes.

Directions : Wash hands, then wash lemons and slice then remove all seeds. Squeeze in water in a jug. Add stevia, and sweeten to taste, then add ice cubes. So refreshing, and can be served all year round. Lemons have *Vitamin C* and it will help keep your immune system strong. *Natural Stevia sugar*, has low glycemic index, which makes it good for diabetics and those wanting to lose weight, and of course for all children, prevents cavities and it also boosts the immune system.

Home-Made Trail Mix by Stephanie Grey

Ingredients : Use your favorite nuts and dried fruits like unsalted nuts, walnuts, sunflower or pumpkin seeds. Add dried apples, pineapple, cherries, apricots or raisins and also whole grain cereals to the mix.

Directions : Place in small zip lock bags , close and shake ingredients together.

Blueberry Smoothie by Stephanie Grey

Ingredients : Blend 1 cup frozen strawberries, 1 cup frozen banana and ½-1 cup apple juice or frozen yogurt.

Directions : Serve right away. Mmm so good and so healthy!!

You can also refreeze in ice cubes with toothpicks. Be creative!

Sweet Potato Fries by Stephanie Grey

Ingredients : 2 medium sweet potatoes, cut into wedges, ½ tsp. grounded ginger, 1/8 tsp. of cinnamon, 1/4 tsp. ground cumin, 1/8 tsp. black pepper and salt, 1/4 tsp. garlic powder , Vegetable oil spray.

Directions **:** Combine sweet potatoes, cinnamon, salt, cumin, black pepper and garlic powder in a plastic bag, seal and shake. Place on a baking sheet coated with vegetable spray. Bake for about 20 minutes, flipping them during cooking. Serve with natural ketchup (see below).

Going Green for Ketchup by Stephanie Grey

Ingredients : 1 chopped tomato,1 tbsp. fresh garlic, fresh basil leaves

3 dates pitted,¼ cup extra virgin olive oil, dash of salt,1-2 tbsp. Apple Cider Vinegar,

Directions : Blend all together to a paste.

*****Remember food safety guidelines, especially washing of hands after handling raw meat or produce and also washing of hands before eating. Put your kids in charge, let them name a new vegetable or fruit and arrange them in a fun design or shape. So after eating all these healthy fruits and vegetables, which are great for dental health, lets go *" Brush Up on Healthy Teeth."* (CDC, 2013). ******Caution : Remember parents or caregivers of children, know each child's allergies and if possible they should wear a wrist band with same. Food allergies can be deadly, and know the ingredients of the foods your child will eat !!

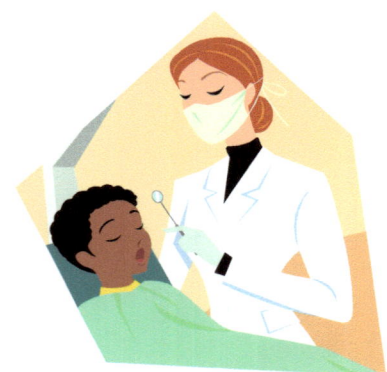

<u>Simple Steps for Kids Smiles</u>

1. Start cleaning teeth early in life!

2. Use the right amount of fluoride toothpaste!

3. Supervise brushing !

4. Talk to your child's doctor or dentist !

****Early care for your children's teeth will protect their smile and their health. Also, making sure they brush their teeth after meals and before bed-time, will help preserve their smile for years to come!!**

Chapter 6 : Spanish /Mexican Recipes !!

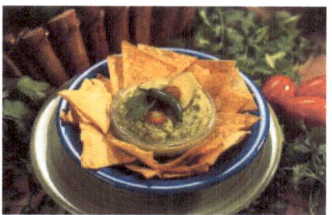

Gazpacho Sevillano

Ingredients : 1 small clove garlic, peeled, ¼ small green pepper, ½ small onion

2 large ripe tomatoes, ¼ small cucumber, 6 tbsp. olive oil

2 tbsp. vinegar, 4 cups ice water, dash of salt.

Directions : Crush garlic, pepper cut in strips, onion, and salt. Add tomato and cucumber and mash. Gradually stir in oil and strain into a deep bowl. Pour in cups of ice water, add salt to taste, mix well and serve cold. Serve with diced cucumber, green pepper, chopped tomato and whole grain croutons, but serve apart for each person.

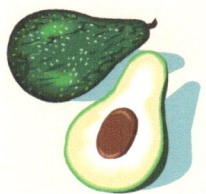

Guacamole

1 large ripe avocado, 1 tsp. lemon, 2 Tbsp. reduced fat sour cream,

1 fresh tomato, chopped, ½ cup grated carrots, pepper to taste.

Cut avocado in half and peel it, throw away the seed. Mix in tomatoes and pepper and then sprinkle with grated carrots. Serve on pita bread or whole grain crackers. Allow your kids to help with preparing this great Mexican dish.

Turkey Tacos

Ingredients : 1-2 pounds of turkey mince, organic preferred, Dash of salt and pepper, Chopped onions- 1 medium red or 2 escallion shoots, 1 tsp. cayenne pepper, 1 tsp. paprika, 1 head of green lettuce chopped, ½ pound of shredded Mexican cheese, ½ cup of guacamole (see recipe above!) , 1 package of corn tacos. *Directions* : Warm tacos in oven at 350 degrees until crisp, do not burn and remove. Cook turkey after mixing with spices above, except lettuce and Mexican Cheese. Place chopped lettuce and cooked turkey in taco shells, then add guacamole on top. Serve with beverage of choice, good for parties, Sunday/Saturday dinners or any day, like at football games!

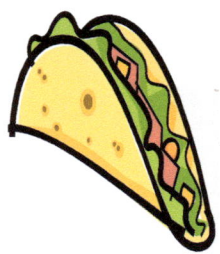

All these are my favorite recipes I make when I want to enjoy Mexico and Spanish foods, which I love! Also attend events like International Fairs, Mexican/Spanish events and learn about their culture, Taco Bell serves some foods and area restaurants, just remember portions, especially if you're a diabetic or have weight problems.

Chapter 7 : Vegetarian Recipes

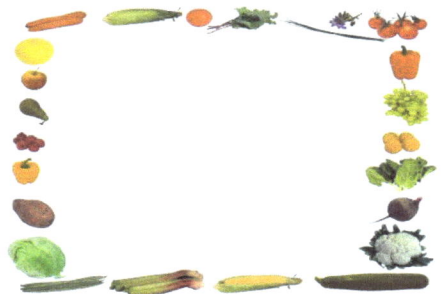

The vegetarian diet has been around long before Noah's flood, and it resulted in many living for long years with very few illnesses. It's been proven to be very healthy and reduces the incidence of diseases, leading to better quality of life. Some people eat some days without meat or during fasts, like the Daniel Fasts which eliminates meat and depends on plant proteins as their source of proteins. Many dietary programs now promote eating of more fruits and vegetables and limiting meats, and also increasing grains. I personally, choose some days as *"Meatless Days",* and experiment with vegetables, fruits, sauces, dressings and its really amazing, how delicious they can be.

Tomato Soup

Ingredients : 2 tbsp. butter, 1 onion chopped, 1 clove garlic, 2 lbs. plum tomatoes cut in halves, 1 cup tomato paste, 2 tbsp. chopped basil and 2 tbsp. chopped parsley.

Direction : Heat butter and sauté onion and garlic until softened, then add tomatoes and tomato paste, then basil. Cover and cook for 15 minutes and then strain to remove tomato skin and seeds and warm again, then add parsley as garnish. Serve with whole grain bread toasted or croutons or crackers. Nice for winter or cold days!

Banana-Pineapple Smoothie

Ingredients : 1 cup yogurt, 6 medium strawberries, 1 cup crushed pineapple with juice, 1 medium banana, 1 tsp. vanilla and 4 ice cubes. Blend until pureed and smooth and serve right away. Lots of Potassium, fiber, protein and low in fat! Great for those trying to lose weight!

Pinto Bean Burgers by Stephanie Grey

Ingredients : 1 can pinto beans or cooked, 3 tbsp. minced onion, dash of salt, 1 tsp. chili powder, 1 ½ tsp. parsley, 1/3 cup flower.

Directions : Mix together, form patties and fry in very little olive oil. Serve on whole grain buns, with lettuce, tomato, mustard and other toppings that are low calorie. Watch the mayonnaise-high in fat! Enjoy ! (Beans can be substituted with black or garbanzo beans).

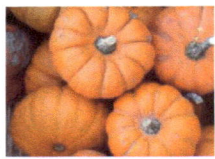

Pumpkin & Pepitas (Pumpkin Seeds) Recipes

Did you know pumpkin seeds hold a tremendous amount of nutrients good for your body, and are very easy to use in recipes or eat toasted. Some people dry them and eat them raw! The next time you buy a pumpkin, all parts can be eaten. The skin when cooked becomes very soft and so delicious, and then you can also make soup and pies, by blending. The seeds, can be washed to remove mesh, and then dry. Toast lightly and add cinnamon and sugar or eat them as is!

The health benefits are: prostate protection, improved bladder function, depression (contains l-tryptophan), prevention of osteoporosis, natural inflammatory, prevent kidney stones, treatment of parasites, great source of magnesium—1/2 cup gives you 92 mg daily!, lowers cholesterol and prevents cancer due to phytosterols. High amount of potassium (1044mg in 1 cup), 39 gm of protein (78% RDA), high in iron and fiber (32%). So what are you waiting for? Go scoop those pumpkin seeds, wash and dry them, then toast. Enjoy!

Herbed Potatoes

Ingredients : 6 large red potatoes, washed and sliced thin, 3 tbsp. fresh rosemary, chopped fine, 2 tbsp. extra virgin olive oil, dash of salt and pepper. Preheat oven to 375 degrees and place all ingredients on a cookie sheet and toss to coat. Bake in oven for 15 minutes or until crisp. Serve immediately. High in protein and fiber.

Source : Church Health Center Wellness Education, visit **www.chreader.org** for more recipes.

Chick Pea Salad

Ingredients : 1 can chick peas low sodium, rinsed and drained, 1 medium red or yellow pepper chopped 1 medium red onion chopped, 1 tbsp. of balsamic vinegar, 2 tbps. of extra virgin olive oil, ¼ tsp. garlic powder and ginger-grounded, dash of salt and pepper.

Directions : Mix all together, chill for 20 minutes and then serve with favorite meat and beverage. Great for summer barbeques!

Chapter 8 : Exercise & Foot Care Recipes by Stephanie Grey

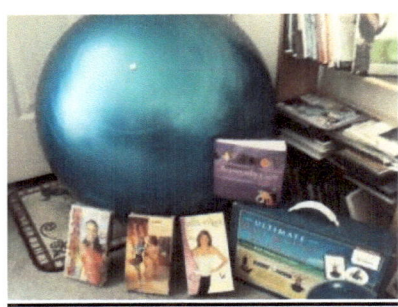

Along with healthy eating, comes being physically active, and everyone needs to have a personal fitness plan, which can be done at home, in community or on the job. Here's some general information about exercise and you can tailor it to meet your own specific, unique needs. A fitness plan has various components, which are:

- *Warm Up (5-10 minutes before each exercise session)*

- *Muscular Strength (20 minutes 2-3 times a week)*

- *Muscular endurance (20 minutes 2-3 days a week)*

- *Cardio-Respiratory endurance: (30-60 minutes 5 times a week. The 30-60 minutes can be broken up into 15-30 minute intervals twice a day).*

- *Flexibility/Stretching : (15-20 minutes a day)*

- *Cool down (5-10 minutes after each exercise session)*

Other aspects of developing a fitness plan are:

- Waist/Hip Ratio : divide your waist by your hip measurement

Values :

Male	Female	Health Risk Based Solely on WHR
0.95 or below	0.80 or below	Low Risk
0.96 to 1.0	0.81 to 0.85	Moderate Risk
1.0+	0.85+	High Risk

***Take your picture before your program then again in six months.

Thigh measurements : Right _____Left_____

Labs : Fasting Blood Glucose _____

Cholesterol_____

Blood Pressure_____

Resting Heart Rate_____

Target Heart Rate_____

Maximum Heart Rate_____

***Here's how you calculate your Maximum

Heart Rate Range!

Take your age and subtract from 220 then for lower level multiply by 55% (.55) or higher level multiply by 90% (.90). The lower HR level is used for burning fat and the higher level for cardiovascular fitness. **Example** : I am 49 years old, so lower level is 220-49 X 55 = 94.05 and higher level is :   220-49 x 90% = 154.

Hydration : Divide your weight by 2, that is the amount of water you need daily. Let's say you weigh 180 pounds, then you need 90 ounces of water a day, about 9 - 10 ozs. eight times a day.

*****Precaution for those with chronic diseases : Please consult your physician for guidelines on how to exercise,   we are not doctors and do not prescribe treatments.

We are only a support system for you to share with your physicians. *****

Recipe for Foot Care by Stephanie Grey

As you enhance your wellness, wearing proper foot wear, is just as important as what you eat. Many foot injuries from those who work out, comes from people not wearing the right foot gear and also not taking care of their feet. If you are a diabetic then your doctor should refer you to a Podiatrist, but you still have to know what to do at home. One can get injury to their knees, shin, ankle, heel and foot, so you should examine same each day. After your bath is a good time and learn to massage your feet often and examine the skin.

Plantar Fasciitis is a common heel problem caused by improper foot wear, and plantar fascia is where the connective tissue that connects the balls of the feet to the heel gets inflamed from repeated stress. The symptoms are burning or aching pain in the heel of the foot. One should get an orthotic to support your arch and heel. Did you know, as your foot gets injured it can cause knee and hip pain, and ultimately those areas feet damaged as well. So, get proper footwear, so your workout routine will remain " *injury-free* ".

Diabetics!!: You should examine your feet daily after each bath and look for cuts or open areas, because nerve damage can cause you not to feel pain. Many diabetics have lost their feet by amputation from gangrene. Foot exercises daily as per md order, and sometimes the podiatrists have to cut your nails.

Chapter 9 : Cancer Prevention Tips

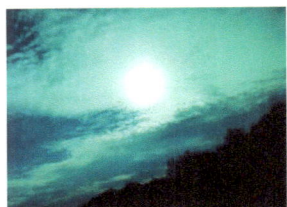

1. Apply sunscreen every-day, even on cloudy days with a SPF of about 30 or more.

2. Seek shade, especially during the hours of 10 am and 4 pm.

3. If you are near water , sand or snow, the reflection intensifies the damaging rays of the sun, leading to increased risk for sunburns as well.

4. Get adequate amounts of Vitamin D, through food and/or supplements, not from sun alone.

5. Avoid tanning beds, as they can cause damage just as from natural sunlight, very deceiving.

6. Do your own skin assessment , and use a mirror for your back. Look for moles and skin changes, report to your doctor early, skin cancer can be cured.

7. Those who have jobs on the road and exposed to sun constantly need to have their sunscreen and apply it ongoing throughout the day, or they can have severe skin damage.

8. Cover up, wear loose fitting clothes and also UV-protected sunglasses and wide rimmed hats to cover your eyes, ears, scalp and neck.

9. Maintain adequate weight through exercise and healthy nutrition, visit **American Cancer Society** *(www.cancer.org)* and **American Institute of Cancer Research** *(www.aicr.org)* for more information.

10. ***Caution for children!! :*** Children's skin is very sensitive and the critical period when UV radiation can do the most damage in just a few minutes. It can cause burns which can have

permanent damage. Parents or caregivers should apply sunscreen 20 minutes before exposure with SPF of 15 and can block 93% of UV rays. Encourage children and youth to play in the shade and wear hats or caps. Provide them with sunglasses to protect eyes and clothing should be light weight , long-sleeved shirts and pants-for those with increased sensitivity to sunlight. Be a good role model as well and practice sun-safety, then your child and youth will follow!!

11. Quit smoking and avoid second hand smoke, especially in your home, and also protect your children from second hand smoke !!

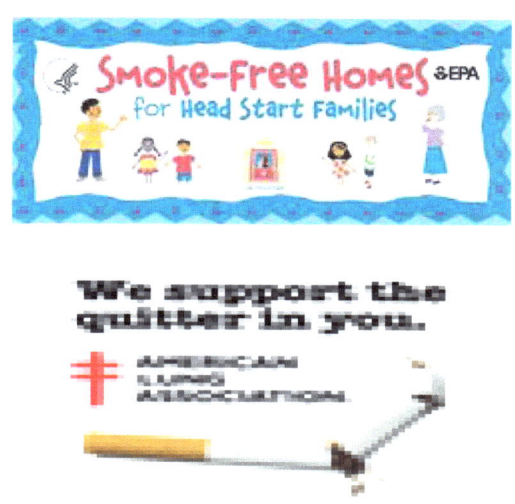

12. Drink a lot of water to flush toxins out , especially good for bladder and colon cancer prevention.

13. Eat many fruits and vegetables, which in antioxidants which will remove free radicals, which cause cancer. *Wash your fruits and vegetables with white vinegar and water (1:3), to remove waxes and pesticides, especially those which are non-organic !!*

14. Filter your water from taps and use non-toxic cleaning agents like white vinegar and water , or lemon oil and water.

15. Make sure your home has adequate ventilation and clean air, especially from outside car pollution and also clean your automobiles with non-toxic cleaning agents, and change your car filter for air, at each car service. Place air-purifying green plants throughout your home, to keep air clean, but watch for mold, especially in winter months.

16. Manage stressors and practice relaxation exercises daily, as too much stress creates more free radicals, and will increase your risk for cancer.

Recipe for Sleep by Rosemary Aslund

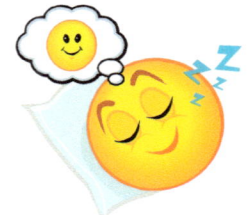

Ingredients:

1 banana, dash of cinnamon,

1 tsp. vanilla extract,

milk of your choice.

Directions : Blend until smooth and drink before bedtime. Natural sleep medicine, non-addicting, leaves you rested in the morning!

10 : My Favorite Natural Home - Cleaning Recipes

White Vinegar & Water

White Vinegar is a must for any home, as it has many uses, not just for cooking. Here's some ways to use white vinegar. Mix one part white vinegar to three parts water, and use to clean floors, counter tops, bathrooms, toilet bowls, bathtub film, unclog showerhead, clean shower curtain, dishwashers and laundry. Also use to wash fruits and vegetables, getting rid of dirt, wax and pesticides. Remove mold and mildew from window seals and bathroom curtains.

Lemon Oil & Water:

This is made from lemon peel, and has many uses. Used in skin and hair care, respiratory tract infections, fatigue, antiseptic and aromatherapy. Can be used also to purify the air.

Ingredients : 8 drops lemon oil, 1 drop clove oil, 2 drops thyme oil and 1 drop tea tree oil.

Directions : Mix together and heat them in a diffuser. Cleans and disinfects stale air in the home.

General cleaning : To clean home, just add 10 drops to a gallon of water and put in a spray bottle. Keep away from your eyes !!

Did You Know, Green Plants can clean your air in your home??

Placing *Green Plants* through out your home, also helps to clean the air, especially in the winter months, when you keep windows closed many times. Opening your window at least for an hour each day, even during winter will also help keep your air clean. Watch the plants for mold and water as needed and ask your local nursery for plants used for cleaning air in homes. Clean air, helps to reduce allergies and helps fight colds and flus in winter months!

Chapter 11 : Recipes for healthy hearts and minds !!

We couldn't finish without these recipes for your heart and mind, where all we do, think or say, begins. We all are faced with many stressors daily, and we need a plan to face same proactively versus reactively. Many have faced traumatic situations in their life, but we have to develop a plan to cope. One hat doesn't fit all, so you have to be patient as you heal, in God's timing. I learnt to use scriptures, when negative thoughts emerge, and it's really a process, but here's some good ones:

" God has not given us a spirit of fear, but of power,

love and a sound mind. "

"Beloved, we wish above all things that you all prosper

and be in health, even as your soul prospereth.

" We can do all things, through Christ who

strengthens us. "

Forgiveness is also healing, and doesn't mean you accept what people may have done to you, but you have learnt to *" Let go, and let God."*

The Bible says :

" Bear with each other and forgive whatever

grievances you may have against each other.

Forgive as the Lord forgave you. "

If Jesus forgave others, then if we say we follow Him, then we too must forgive. We don't forget the harm, and will be wise in not being harmed by those people again, but forgiveness is a healing process, which will heal you and give you peace. Un-forgiveness, can also lead to many physical ailments, like ulcers, heart disease and stress – related problems as well. There are really many more, but God's Word is healing and helps you feel closer to Him each day.

Here's some cool *Stress Management Tips* you need to practiced, weekly or when you face stressful times.

1. ***Take time to enjoy nature*** and go for walks, or visit the beach, mountains, gardens and river sides. Have a fitness buddy- your spouse, mate, children or trusted friend, who also loves to exercise. Join a walking group at your Church, in your community or with neighbors. Use music, like natural sounds of the ocean, along with your walks or periods of meditation.

2. ***Seek professional help*** if you cannot handle life's stressors, and sometimes you need medicines. I take medicines, along with seeing a psychiatrist, coupled with my prayer times, bible studies and fellowshipping with faith based believers. Sometimes, there's stigma and people are afraid to seek help but its more expensive when you don't, and your life won't have the best quality.

3. ***Get a hobby*** you like and join a network that shares that hobby, like I am a writer and learn from other writers through networking with writing groups. I also like dancing , which there is a variety to choose from. Other hobbies are : exercise, art, music, knitting and many more, like gardening. Community gardens are common and can be fun, and volunteering in your community, can open you up to doors of friends and opportunities.

4. ***Address your spirituality***, it will help you deal with any mental or physical challenge you may be experiencing. So much trauma around and depressing events, but drawing close to God, understanding your true purpose in life, will help you use your gifts, talents and experiences to serve those He has called you to lead.

Thanks!!

Be Healthy Ministries, Inc. thanks every one for their support of our books, geared at promoting health, preventing illnesses, and keeping the public safe, especially in these challenging times. May God bless you always.

Contact Information : Stephanie Grey Director/RN

Be Healthy Ministries, Inc., 252-702-0861

snursegrey@aol.com, www.behealthyministries.com

Twitter : @behealthy

Facebook : facebook.com/snursegrey

Products

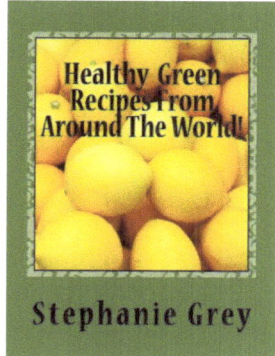 For additional copies of this book, please order at

www.createspace.com/4353175

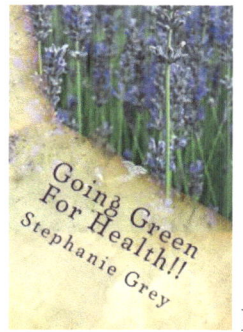 Please visit **www.createspace.com/3951499** to order or search

Amazon.com.

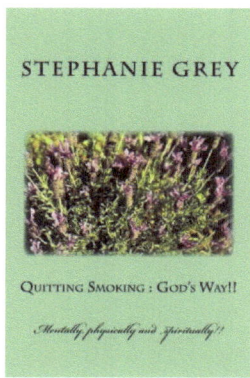 Please visit **www.createspace.com/3575316** to order or search

Amazon.com.

Thanks for your support !!